T0233205

Cambridge Elements ≡

Elements in Molecular Oncology
edited by
Edward P. Gelmann
University of Arizona

EGFR-DIRECTED THERAPY IN LUNG CANCER

So Yeon Kim
Yale School of Medicine

Daniel B. Costa
Harvard Medical School

Daisuke Shibahara
Harvard Medical School

Susumu Kobayashi
Harvard Medical School

Balazs Halmos
Albert Einstein College of Medicine

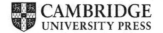
CAMBRIDGE
UNIVERSITY PRESS

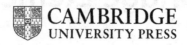

CAMBRIDGE
UNIVERSITY PRESS

Shaftesbury Road, Cambridge CB2 8EA, United Kingdom

One Liberty Plaza, 20th Floor, New York, NY 10006, USA

477 Williamstown Road, Port Melbourne, VIC 3207, Australia

314–321, 3rd Floor, Plot 3, Splendor Forum, Jasola District Centre,
New Delhi – 110025, India

103 Penang Road, #05–06/07, Visioncrest Commercial, Singapore 238467

Cambridge University Press is part of Cambridge University Press & Assessment,
a department of the University of Cambridge.

We share the University's mission to contribute to society through the pursuit of
education, learning and research at the highest international levels of excellence.

www.cambridge.org
Information on this title: www.cambridge.org/9781009342308

DOI: 10.1017/9781009342285

© So Yeon Kim, Daniel B. Costa, Daisuke Shibahara, Susumu Kobayashi, and Balazs
Halmos 2023

This publication is in copyright. Subject to statutory exception and to the provisions
of relevant collective licensing agreements, no reproduction of any part may take
place without the written permission of Cambridge University Press & Assessment.

First published 2023

A catalogue record for this publication is available from the British Library.

ISBN 978-1-009-34230-8 Paperback
ISSN 2634-7490 (online)
ISSN 2634-7482 (print)

Additional resources for this publication at www.cambridge.org/EGFR.

Cambridge University Press & Assessment has no responsibility for the persistence
or accuracy of URLs for external or third-party internet websites referred to in this
publication and does not guarantee that any content on such websites is, or will
remain, accurate or appropriate.

Every effort has been made in preparing this Element to provide accurate and up-to-
date information that is in accord with accepted standards and practice at the time of
publication. Although case histories are drawn from actual cases, every effort has been
made to disguise the identities of the individuals involved. Nevertheless, the authors,
editors, and publishers can make no warranties that the information contained herein
is totally free from error, not least because clinical standards are constantly changing
through research and regulation. The authors, editors, and publishers therefore
disclaim all liability for direct or consequential damages resulting from the use of
material contained in this Element. Readers are strongly advised to pay careful
attention to information provided by the manufacturer of any drugs or equipment
that they plan to use.

EGFR-Directed Therapy in Lung Cancer

Elements in Molecular Oncology

DOI: 10.1017/9781009342285
First published online: January 2023

So Yeon Kim
Yale School of Medicine

Daniel B. Costa
Harvard Medical School

Daisuke Shibahara
Harvard Medical School

Susumu Kobayashi
Harvard Medical School

Balazs Halmos
Albert Einstein College of Medicine

Author for correspondence: Balazs Halmos, bahalmos@montefiore.org

Abstract: Epidermal growth factor receptor (*EGFR*)-mutant non-small cell lung cancer (NSCLC) is a clinically important driver alteration affecting approximately 15–30% of lung cancer patients worldwide. Treatments for *EGFR*-Exon 19 deletion and Exon 21 L858R NSCLC have evolved over the last decade, from first-generation reversible tyrosine kinase inhibitors (TKI) to third-generation irreversible TKIs, of which osimertinib has been widely accepted as first-line therapy. Despite survival improvement seen with osimertinib and its efficacy against acquired T790M mutation, resistance through on-target and off-target pathways eventually develops. This Element describes the structural biology and pathophysiology of *EGFR*-mutant NSCLC and discusses past, current, and future treatment options in the metastatic, neoadjuvant, and adjuvant settings. It also describes the biology and recently approved treatment for *EGFR*-Exon 20 insertion mutation and the treatment for the uncommon Exon 18 (G719X), 20 (S768I), and 21 (L861Q) mutations. In addition, it outlines the promising clinical applications of circulating tumor DNA (ctDNA).

Keywords: non-small cell lung cancer, EGFR, immunotherapy, resistance mechanisms, osimertinib

© So Yeon Kim, Daniel B. Costa, Daisuke Shibahara, Susumu Kobayashi, and Balazs Halmos 2023

ISBNs: 9781009342308 (PB), 9781009342285 (OC)
ISSNs: 2634-7490 (online), 2634-7482 (print)

Contents

Further online supplementary material for Table 1 can be
accessed at www.cambridge.org/EGFR.

1 Structural Biology and Mechanism of Activation of *EGFR*

Identified in 1978, epidermal growth factor receptor (EGFR) is a 170 kDa membrane protein, belonging to the erythroblastic leukemia viral oncogene homolog (ERBB) family of four related receptors: EGFR/HER1/ERBB-1, HER2/ERBB-2/NEU, HER3/ERBB-3, and HER4/ERBB-4 [1]. Each family member is composed of an extracellular domain (subdivided into four domains (I–IV): a transmembrane domain, an intracellular tyrosine kinase domain (consisting of an N-lobe and a C-lobe), and a C-terminal domain. Binding of ligands such as epidermal growth factor (EGF) and transforming growth factor-α (TGF-α) to EGFR induces homodimerization and heterodimerization with ERBB-2, ERBB-3, and ERBB-4 receptors through interactions between extracellular domains. The ligands bind to two distinct sites (subdomains I and III) within the same receptor molecule and induce conformational changes in the extracellular region of EGFR, enabling subdomain II to facilitate homo- and heterodimerization [2]. Dimerization of the extracellular regions of EGFR allosterically activates the intracellular tyrosine kinase domain (TKD) by direct interface between the C-lobe of one TKD and the N-lobe of another TKD [3]. The activated TKD triggers autophosphorylation of various tyrosine residues of the C-terminal domain, allowing coupling with intracellular downstream signaling proteins, and activation of several signaling pathways, including RAS/RAF/MAPK, PI3 K/Akt/mTOR, STAT, and BIM/cyclin D/DUSP pathways (described in the following subsections), inducing cell growth, proliferation, differentiation, migration, inhibition of apoptosis, and regulation of cell growth.

RAS/RAF/MAPK

Following the autophosphorylation of the kinase domain, adaptor proteins such as Src homology 2 domain-containing (Shc) and growth factor receptor-bound protein 2 (GRB2) are recruited. GRB2 is activated through direct phosphorylation of EGFR or through phosphorylated Shc and on activation, GRB2 binds to Son of Sevenless (SOS). The GRB2-SOS complex then leads to initiation of the RAS/RAF/MAPK pathway [4, 5, 6]. Activated rat sarcoma (RAS) in turn activates rapidly accelerated fibrosarcoma (RAF) and the downstream pathway mitogen-activated protein kinases (MAPK), which results in cell proliferation, survival, migration, and angiogenesis [7].

PI3 K/Akt/mTOR

Activated EGFR also interacts with GRB2-associated binding protein 1 (GAB1), which results in recruitment of phosphatidylinositol 3-kinase

(PI3 K) and subsequent activation of serine/threonine protein kinase (Akt) and the mammalian target of rapamycin (mTOR). The PI3 K/Akt/mTOR pathway has been demonstrated to be activated early in lung carcinogenesis and regulates cellular apoptosis, invasion, metabolism, and cell growth [8].

STAT

The signal transducer and activator of transcription 3 protein (STAT3), which is phosphorylated and activated by EGFR, forms homodimers (STAT3/STAT3) or heterodimers (STAT3/STAT1). STAT3-dimers translocate into the nucleus and activate the expression of specific target genes [9].

BIM/Cyclin D/DUSP

BIM, a BCL2 homology domain 3 (BH3)-only proapoptotic protein (also known as BCL2-like 11), is regulated by extracellular signal-regulated kinase (ERK) MAPK pathways, resulting in inhibition of cell death in EGFR-mutant non-small cell lung cancer (NSCLC) [10]. Cyclin D1 is a key downstream effector of EGFR signaling, which promotes cell cycle G1/S transition [11]. Dual-specificity MAPK phosphatases (DUSP), which are activated by the MAPK pathway, dampen MAPK signaling as a key negative feedback control of EGFR signaling [12, 13, 14].

2 Epidemiology of *EGFR*-Mutant Lung Cancer

EGFR mutations are present in approximately 10%–15% of patients with Caucasian or African ancestry, with a higher prevalence, of up to 50%, seen in patients with Asian ancestry, more frequently among women, younger patients, and nonsmokers [15, 16, 17]. Differential prevalence among the Asian population is also observed, with a higher frequency of up to 65% seen in patients of Vietnamese descent [15]. While adenocarcinoma is the most common histology associated with *EGFR* mutations (odds ratio (OR) 4.1, 95% confidence interval (CI) 3.6–4.8), mutations have been observed in mixed adenosquamous histology and rarely in squamous cell (typically in nonsmokers) and small cell cancers, which typically presents as a transformation from *EGFR*-mutant NSCLC [17, 18, 19]. Because of this differential histologic association, the European Society of Medical Oncology (ESMO) guidelines recommend *EGFR* biomarker testing in metastatic NSCLC patients with only nonsquamous NSCLC, but due to the increased frequency of *EGFR* mutations in non- or former light smokers, *EGFR* mutation testing should be expanded to include patients with mixed or squamous cell histology in patients with no or light smoking history and in patients whose sampling was limited and thus mixed histology cannot be entirely excluded [17, 20, 21]. Though rarer, *EGFR* mutations in patients with a heavy smoking history have also been observed, and the National Comprehensive Cancer Network (NCCN) guidelines recommend *EGFR* biomarker testing as part of expanded molecular profiling in all patients diagnosed with metastatic NSCLC [15, 22, 23].

3 *EGFR*-Associated Oncogenesis

Oncogenic activation of EGFR has been postulated to occur through multiple mechanisms and include overactivation of EGFR, overexpression of EGFR, and somatic mutations in the intracellular TKD. Ligands of EGFR, such as EGF and TGF-α, are frequently expressed in NSCLC, and lead to receptor hyperactivity by an autocrine loop [24]. Approximately 60% of NSCLC are also observed to have overexpression of EGFR through gene amplification, which occurs in about 15% of adenocarcinoma and 30% of squamous cell carcinoma [25, 26, 27].

Mutations that are the only fully validated oncogenic aberrations with current therapeutic implications occur in the active site of the TKD and serve to disrupt autoinhibitory interactions with the ATP-binding pocket, leading to ligand-independent constitutive activation of the kinase domain [28]. Approximately 90% of common *EGFR* mutations consist of in-frame deletions in Exon 19 or substitutions of leucine for arginine at codon 858 (L858 R) in Exon 21 of the *EGFR* gene [29, 30]. *EGFR* Exon 20 insertion mutations represent the third most common *EGFR* mutations, amounting to 6%–12% of pathogenic *EGFR* alteration [31, 32]. Their analysis requires detailed sequencing, since the subtype p.A763_Y764insFQEA mimics a structural change akin to Exon 21 L861Q, and is sensitive to first-, second-, and third-generation tyrosine kinase inhibitors (TKIs), whereas other insertion types are generally resistant to standard doses of these agents [33, 34]. Other uncommon mutations include point mutations at amino acids in Exon 18 (G719X), Exon 20 (S768I), and Exon 21 (L861Q), and compound mutations [31, 35, 36]. Treatment response and prognosis of cancers with Exon 20 insertions have been poor until the recent approval of amivantamab-vmjw and mobocertinib, which are administered in the second-line setting after progression on platinum-based chemotherapy [37, 38, 39]. Other uncommon non-Exon 20 insertions may confer sensitivity to the second-generation EGFR TKI, afatinib, which is FDA approved for this indication; however, activity with third-generation agents has also been demonstrated (**Figure 1**) [36, 39, 40, 41, 42].

4 Tyrosine Kinase Inhibitors (TKIs) as Targeted Treatment for *EGFR*-Mutant NSCLC

First-Generation TKI: Gefitinib and Erlotinib

EGFR-activating mutations are heterogeneous, and the approved use of TKIs has been guided by biochemical specificity (**Figure 1**). TKIs inhibit activation of

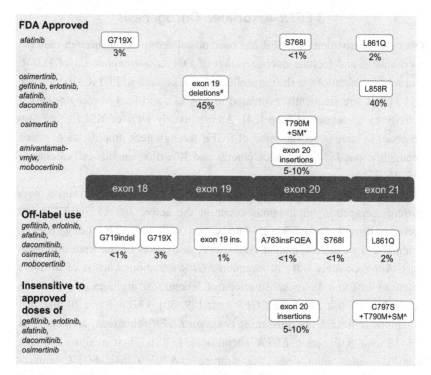

Figure 1 Prevalence of *EGFR* tyrosine kinase domain mutations in lung cancer and associated FDA-approved therapies.

Notes: FDA = Food and Drug Administration.

SM = sensitizing mutation.

X in G719X = substitution for several different amino acids and is not a stop codon. Approved doses of TKIs are: gefitinib 250 mg daily, erlotinib 150 mg daily (first-generation TKIs); afatinib 40 mg daily (second-generation TKI); dacomitinib 45 mg daily (second-generation TKI); osimertinib 80 mg daily (third-generation TKI); mobocertinib 160 mg daily (Exon 20 active TKI).

\# Most common Exon 19 deletion is delE746_A750 (LREA motif).

* Cause of acquired resistance to gefitinib, erlotinib, and afatinib in more than 50%.

^ Cause of osimertinib resistance in approximately 10%–30%.

Other types of EGFR aberrations that lead to downstream activation (kinase domain duplications and kinase fusions) are not depicted. The figure was adapted from Y. Sheikine, D. Rangachari, D. C. McDonald et al., Clin Lung Cancer; **17**(6):483. (2016).

EGFR-associated oncogenesis by competitively blocking the binding of adenosine triphosphate (ATP) to the intracellular tyrosine kinase pocket of the receptor [43]. The majority of translational and clinical research has focused on the most prevalent *EGFR* kinase domain mutations – *EGFR* Exon 19 indels and Exon 21-L858 R. Gefitinib, a reversible first-generation EGFR TKI, demonstrated efficacy in 2009 in the landmark phase 3 trial (IPASS), which randomized metastatic treatment-naïve Asian patients with advanced lung adenocarcinoma who had a limited smoking history to gefitinib versus platinum-based chemotherapy, and demonstrated superior median progression-free survival (PFS) with gefitinib in patients positive for an *EGFR* mutation, and inferior median PFS in patients with wild-type *EGFR* [44]. Following the IPASS study, gefitinib was prospectively evaluated against chemotherapy in patients with metastatic *EGFR*-mutant adenocarcinoma and demonstrated superior PFS, but without overall survival (OS) benefit, possibly due to a high rate of treatment crossover among trial participants [45, 46, 47]. A follow-up post hoc analysis of the IPASS study in 2011 demonstrated *EGFR* to be a predictive biomarker for treatment response to gefitinib, helping launch the field of precision oncology and prompting the wide introduction of biomarker testing in metastatic lung adenocarcinoma [44, 48]. Gefitinib obtained FDA approval in July, 2015, for the management of advanced EGFR-mutated NSCLC, after its demonstrated single-arm efficacy among Caucasian patients in the Iressa Follow-up Measure (IFUM) trial [49]. Erlotinib, a pharmacokinetically similar first-generation TKI, was also FDA approved in May, 2013, for first-line treatment in *EGFR*-mutant metastatic adenocarcinoma based on improved PFS compared to platinum-based doublet chemotherapy [50, 51]. Both drugs had been approved more broadly for the management of advanced NSCLC, but these approvals were rescinded as a better understanding was gained of the clinical utility of these compounds. Both gefitinib and erlotinib are fairly well tolerated oral agents with similar toxicities, such as acneiform skin rash and diarrhea related to wild-type *EGFR* inhibition.

Second-Generation TKI: Afatinib, Dacomitinib

Though first-generation TKI treatments demonstrated favorable efficacy compared to conventional chemotherapies [29, 47, 50, 51, 52], the appearance of drug-resistant clones, such as those with the common T790M gatekeeper mutation, were not unexpected [53, 54]. Second- and third-generation TKIs developed to overcome drug resistance have the capacity to bind covalently to the C797 site of EGFR. Afatinib and dacomitinib, second-generation TKIs, irreversibly inhibit multiple ERBB receptors, including EGFR, HER2, and HER4 [55, 56]. Afatinib was FDA approved for Exon deletion 19 and L858 R mutant metastatic *EGFR* patients in July, 2013, after its demonstration of superior PFS to platinum-pemetrexed and platinum-gemcitabine in the phase 3 LUX-Lung 3 and LUX-Lung 6 trials [30, 57]. Afatinib treatment resulted in superior median OS compared to platinum doublet chemotherapy only for the Exon 19 *EGFR* mutation subtype. No OS benefit was seen among patients with L858 R mutations [58]. The choice of first- or second-generation TKI was studied in ARCHER 1050, in which dacomitinib was shown to result in superior median OS compared to gefitinib (34.1 months vs. 26.8 months) in either treatment-naïve or relapsed patients [59]. Dacomitinib was approved by the FDA as a first-line agent in September, 2018, for treatment of metastatic NSCLC with either *EGFR* Exon 19 deletion or L858 R mutations. While second-generation EGFR TKIs appear somewhat more effective than first-generation drugs, their use is also associated with accentuated target toxicity due to wild-type *EGFR* inhibition yielding a narrow therapeutic index.

Third-Generation TKIs

While erlotinib, gefitinib, afatinib, and dacomitinib are documented as category 1 recommendations in NCCN guidelines, osimertinib, a third-generation irreversible TKI, which selectively and irreversibly inhibits activating *EGFR* mutations and the common T790M gatekeeper mutation associated with early-generation TKIs, is now the preferred TKI for front-line management [53, 60]. Osimertinib is more potent against L858 R/T790M than the wild-type *EGFR* [60, 61] and was initially approved in November, 2015, for patients with acquired T790M who had progressed on first- or second-generation TKIs based on phase 2 AURA and AURA2 studies, and phase 3 AURA3, which demonstrated superior median PFS with osimertinib compared to platinum-pemetrexed (12.5 months vs. 4.3 months) [62, 63, 64]. The phase 3 FLAURA trial demonstrated superior median PFS of osimertinib compared to first-generation TKIs (18.9 months vs. 10.2 months, HR 0.46) in patients with metastatic NSCLC with *EGFR* Exon 19 deletion or L858 R mutations, supporting FDA approval of osimertinib for use in the first-line setting in April, 2018 [61]. Moreover, an updated analysis of the trial data demonstrated superior median OS (38.6 months for osimertinib vs. 31.8 months for first-generation TKIs), and osimertinib is now the accepted preferred frontline TKI for metastatic adenocarcinoma with common *EGFR* mutations [65].

In addition to osimertinib, multiple third-generation TKIs are undergoing clinical development. Lazertinib, an irreversible EGFR TKI with increased selectivity against wild-type EGFR compared to osimertinib, demonstrated synergistic activity with amivantamab *EGFR*-activating mutations (Exon 19 deletion, L858 R) in the phase 1 CHRYSALIS trial of advanced NSCLC patients with 0–9 prior lines of treatment, with an overall response rate (ORR) of 43.5% [66]. Lazertinib as monotherapy was approved in January, 2021, for use in patients with acquired T790M mutation in South Korea, and its efficacy as monotherapy in the frontline setting is being evaluated against gefitinib in the phase 3 LASER301 trial (NCT04248829). Lazertinib in combination with amivantamab is being compared to osimertinib in the MARIPOSA trial (NCT04487080). In China, the phase 3 AENEAS trial of aumolertinib demonstrated superior median PFS compared to gefitinib (19.3 months vs. 9.9 months), with fewer adverse effects in patients with treatment-naïve advanced *EGFR*-mutant NSCLC (Exon 19 deletion, L858 R) [67]. Aumolertinib is approved in China for use in the second-line setting for patients with acquired T790M mutation. Additional third-generation TKIs in clinical study in the frontline setting include alflutinib (NCT03787992), rezivertinib (NCT03866499), abivertinib (NCT03856697), and befotertinib (NCT04206072) [68].

Combining EGFR TKI and Anti-VEGF Treatment

TKI and anti-vascular endothelial growth factor (VEGF) combinations have been prospectively evaluated and demonstrated superior PFS compared to EGFR TKI monotherapy [69, 70]. For example, in the phase 3 placebo-controlled RELAY trial, combination ramucirumab, a human IgG_1 VEGFR2 antagonist with erlotinib, demonstrated superior median PFS (19.4 months vs. 12.4 months, HR 0.59) compared to erlotinib in treatment-naïve *EGFR*-mutant (Exon 19 deletion or L858 R) metastatic NSCLC [71]. This dual-target strategy was designed to inhibit molecular crosstalk between the EGFR and VEGF pathways, which induces both Ras/Raf/mitogen-activated protein kinase (MEK) and PI3 K/AKT/m-TORC signaling [72]. Moreover, EGFR activation induces hypoxia-inducible factor (HIF-1α) activity that promotes VEGF transcription [72]. Based on the positive outcomes of the phase 3 FLAURA and RELAY trials, combination osimertinib and bevacizumab, an anti-VEGF monoclonal antibody, was evaluated in a phase 1/2 open-label setting and demonstrated a favorable overall response rate of 80% in patients with metastatic *EGFR*-mutant lung cancer (Exon 19 deletion, L858 R, G719S + E709A) with no prior EGFR TKI or VEGF therapy [73]. However, randomized phase 2 trials comparing osimertinib and bevacizumab versus osimertinib as monotherapy failed to demonstrate PFS benefit with the combination arm [74, 75]. To define the clinical relevance of combined receptor inhibition a phase 3 trial is ongoing (NCT04181060).

Combination EGFR TKI and Chemotherapy

The addition of first-generation TKIs to platinum-based chemotherapy was prospectively demonstrated to be beneficial in two randomized phase 3 studies of patients with advanced *EGFR*-mutant NSCLC [76, 77]. In both studies, the TKI–chemotherapy combination arms had higher incidence of adverse events of grade 3 or above, especially hematological toxicities [76, 78]. To extend these observations to third-generation TKIs, the FLAURA2 trial is comparing the efficacy of osimertinib versus osimertinib and platinum-based doublet chemotherapy in untreated *EGFR*-mutant NSCLC (NCT04035486). A safety run-in trial to explore feasibility demonstrated that the combination of osimertinib and chemotherapy was well tolerated [79].

5 EGFR TKIs as Adjuvant or Neoadjuvant Therapy

One can expect TKIs to have more cytostatic than cytocidal activity supported by variable results of trials examining their efficacy as adjuvant therapeutic agents. RADIANT and NCIC CTG BR19 were negative phase 3 studies comparing adjuvant erlotinib to placebo in studies that omitted biomarker selection [80, 81]. The phase 3 ADJUVANT-CTONG study, which included patients with *EGFR*-mutated NSCLC, demonstrated DFS (disease-free survival) benefit, but not an OS benefit, of gefitinib when compared against cisplatin-based chemotherapy [82]. In 2018, the phase 3 ADAURA trial, which randomized patients with stage IB-IIIA nonsquamous lung cancer to adjuvant osimertinib or placebo after resection, demonstrated superior median DFS and central nervous system (CNS)–related DFS compared to placebo (DFS median not reached vs. 27.5 months, HR 0.20) [83]. As a result, osimertinib was approved in December, 2020, for adjuvant therapy of patients with Exon 19 deletion or L858 R mutations. The OS data from ADAURA is not yet mature, and other active EGFR-adjuvant trials, including the phase 3 ALCHEMIST-EGFR (NCT02194738) trial of erlotinib and a phase 3 trial in China with adjuvant icotinib (NCT02448797), a first-generation TKI with efficacy against T790M, are both forthcoming. Osimertinib is also being studied as adjuvant treatment following definitive chemoradiation in patients with unresectable stage III NSCLC in the phase III LAURA trial (NCT03521154), and as neoadjuvant therapy as either monotherapy or with chemotherapy in the NEOADAURA trial (NCT04351555).

6 *EGFR*-Exon 20 Insertion Mutations

EGFR Exon 20 insertion mutations are the third most common *EGFR* mutations in lung cancer, representing 6%–12% of *EGFR* mutations [31, 32]. *EGFR* Exon

20 mutations comprise in-frame insertions within Exon 20, leading to structural changes at the protein level following the regulatory C-helix, that activate autophosphorylation and are usually resistant to the approved EGFR TKIs gefitinib, erlotinib, afatinib, dacomitinib, or osimertinib [34, 84, 85, 86]. There are some exceptions, including *EGFR*-A763_Y764insFQEA, which is sensitive to all classes of approved EGFR TKIs, and *EGFR*-D770>GY, which is sensitive either to afatinib or to dacomitinib [33, 87, 88]. For all other *EGFR* Exon 20 insertion mutations, such as the most common insertions with amino acid positions 769, 770, and 771, novel and specific agents have recently been brought to the clinic [89, 90].

Mobocertinib

The oral EGFR TKI mobocertinib was designed as an EGFR Exon 20 active inhibitor and demonstrated consistent efficacy in preclinical models [86, 91]. Results from the phase I/II study EXCLAIM (NCT02716116) recommended a daily dose of 160 mg that was found to also cause cutaneous, mucosal, gastrointestinal, and, less frequently, cardiac adverse events [92]. Initial efficacy was noted among cases with *EGFR* Exon 20 insertion mutations, and the phase II element of the trial patients was treated with mobocertinib after progression on, at least, platinum-doublet chemotherapy. The ORR was 28% (95% CI, 20%–37%), with a median duration of response of 17.5 months (95% CI, 7.4–20.3), median PFS of 7.3 months (95% CI, 5.5–9.2), and median OS of 24.0 months (95% CI, 14.6–28.8) [92]. Other EGFR TKIs with similar preclinical therapeutic windows undergoing clinical development include poziotinib, CLN-081, and others [93, 94].

Amivantamab-vmjw

Rather than direct tyrosine kinase inhibition, a novel treatment strategy employs the bispecific EGFR-MET antibody amivantamab-vmjw, which has shown activity against a number of preclinical *EGFR*-mutated models [95]. Amivantamab is a human EGFR-MET bispecific antibody, which has two binding sites directed at activating and resistant EGFR-mutant proteins and met proto-oncogene (MET) receptor tyrosine kinase. Blockade of ligand-induced activation by binding to each receptor's extracellular domain and receptor degradation inhibits both EGFR and MET signaling. In addition, amivantamab induces antibody-dependent cellular cytotoxicity (ADCC) by immune effector cells [96]. Amivantamab was first tested in the clinic via the phase I CHRYSALIS study (NCT02609776). The majority of patients receiving the recommended dose (1,050 mg amivantamab, or 1,400 mg if ≥ 80 kg, given once weekly for the first month and then once every two weeks thereafter) had received prior platinum-doublets [37].

The ORR was 40% (95% CI, 29%–51%), with a median duration of response of 11.1 months (95% CI, 6.9–not reached) and median PFS of 8.3 months (95% CI, 6.5–10) [37]. Major adverse events included infusion-related reactions, rash, paronychia, hypokalemia, and diarrhea.

Both mobocertinib and amivantamab are being evaluated as first-line treatment of tumors with *EGFR* Exon 20 insertion mutations. The EXCLAIM-2 study (NCT04129502) is comparing mobocertinib against platinum-doublet chemotherapy. The PAPILLON study (NCT04538664) is evaluating the combination of amivantamab and carboplatin-pemetrexed versus carboplatin-pemetrexed. One clinical challenge not fully addressed is the limited CNS activity of these agents. Further development of EGFR TKIs, anti-EGFR antibodies, the correct sequencing of these agents, and their role in combination should improve the care of *EGFR* Exon 20 insertion-mutated lung cancers over the next decade.

7 Resistance Mechanisms and Therapies in Metastatic Resistant *EGFR*-NSCLC

There are multiple biologic and pharmacokinetic mechanisms of resistance to EGFR-directed therapy. Resistance generally is mediated by a finite number of known mechanisms, but there are likely unknown mechanisms not identified by routine biomarker analysis. Often there are on-target *EGFR* mutations that decrease the affinity of the drug for its target. There are off-target genomic aberrations commonly affecting other driver oncogenes that activate downstream pathways shared with *EGFR* serving to "bypass" the inhibitory effect of the EGFR TKI. Less commonly, the tumor can manifest histologic transdifferentiation that manifests a neuroendocrine phenotype with cells that have epigenetically silenced the expression of *EGFR* [97, 98, 99, 100, 101].

Resistant mutations can be acquired during treatment with first- (gefitinib, erlotinib) or second- (afatinib, dacomitinib) generation TKIs. Prior to approval of osimertinib, more than half of acquired second mutations involved Exon 20 T790M, which induces a steric hinderance in the ATP-binding pocket, reducing drug affinity by a factor of 0.001 and enhancing ATP-binding affinity [17, 97, 102, 103]. The importance of these mutations in the clinic was deemphasized by the widespread adoption of osimertinib as the first-line choice for the majority of cases of metastatic NSCCL with *EGFR* Exon 19 indels and L858 R. Furthermore, concerns about drug tolerability and need for greater central nervous system penetration have shifted recent drug development and clinical trials toward resistance to third-generation EGFR TKIs [104, 105].

Informative studies of drug resistance have analyzed tumor growth in the face of osimertinib treatment of cancers with *EGFR*-T790M mutations [100]. In these cases the presence of on-target *EGFR*-C797S, which alters the binding site of osimertinib to EGFR, was found. Also, off-target amplification of *MET* is the most common actionable bypass alteration, but other driver oncogene amplifications/mutations/rearrangements have been found, including *KRAS, BRAF, RET, ALK,* and *ERBB2* (**Figure 2**) [100, 106, 107, 108]. The heterogeneity of resistance has hampered the rapid clinical development of therapies that are effective after the appearance of osimertinib resistance. In fact, there is no currently accepted evidence-based therapy for patients with *EGFR*-mutated lung cancers that progress on first-line osimertinib. The use of standard platinum-doublet chemotherapy is usually recommended, and IMPower150 has evaluated platinum-doublets with bevacizumab and immune checkpoint inhibitor in the post EGFR TKI setting [109, 110].

A number of clinical trials are addressing the issue of EGFR TKI resistance (**Supplementary Table 1**, available online at www.cambridge.org/EGFR). Phase 3 studies are addressing the use of either platinum-based chemotherapy (FLAURA2) or anti-angiogenic agents (EA5182) in combination with osimertinib to delay the emergence of drug-resistant clones. Prior studies with early-generation EGFR TKI have suggested that these strategies may indeed be effective [71, 76]. Testing the combination of third-generation EGFR TKI with the EGFR-MET bispecific antibody amivantamab (MARIPOSA) is also underway (NCT04487080). Smaller studies, based on preclinical models [111, 112], have attempted dual EGFR TKIs to mitigate *EGFR*-T790M and *EGFR*-C797S [113] or MEK coinhibition to try to avoid multiple off-target mechanisms of resistance (**Supplementary Table 1**). Alternative target pathways such as Wnt/β-catenin inhibition using tegavivint, a novel small molecule inhibitor against transducing beta-like protein one (TBL1), are also being studied in the frontline setting with osimertinib to delay osimertinib resistance (NCT04780568). Trials that explore treatment of patients with osimertinib resistance are also ongoing [100]. Treatment strategies include the use of chemoimmunotherapy (KEYNOTE-789) [114] and the use of continuation osimertinib with chemotherapy (COMPEL) (**Supplementary Table 1**). Two large studies are focusing on specific genetic mechanisms of resistance. The SAVANNAH trial is open for cases with *MET* amplification and the ORCHARD trial for cases with a variety of resistance mechanisms, including *EGFR*-C797S, *EGFR* amplification, *ALK* rearrangement, and *RET* rearrangement (**Supplementary Table 1**). Encouraging data has recently emerged using a combination of EGFR and MET inhibitors (osimertinib plus savolitinib), as reported from the phase I TATTON study [115].

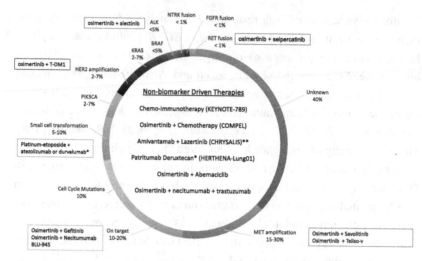

Figure 2 Acquired resistance mutations on osimertinib. Biomarker-specific
   treatments currently undergoing clinical trials are listed aside acquired
resistance mutations. Some of the nonbiomarker-driven treatments undergoing
                clinical trials are listed within the ring.

Notes: * FDA approved.
** Higher overall response rate observed with MET immunohistochemistry positivity.

Additional novel strategies are being tested to overcome TKI resistance, such
as combining EGFR TKI and EGFR-targeting antibodies. Anti-EGFR antibodies competitively bind to extracellular regions of EGFR and promote
internalization and degradation of the antibody-receptor complex, thereby
inhibiting EGFR downstream signaling [116]. The combination of the third-
generation EGFR TKI lazertinib and the bispecific EGFR-MET antibody amivantamab has demonstrated modest clinical activity, with ORR 36%, in patients
who progressed on osimertinib [66, 117]. Patients whose drug resistance was
mediated by *EGFR/MET* had a 47% ORR, whereas patients in whom *EGFR/
MET* was not seen had a 29% ORR. Among 10 patients who had a positive
EGFR/MET by immunohistochemical staining, the ORR with amivantamab
and lazertinib was as high as 90% [117]. A follow-up CHRYSALIS-2 trial
demonstrated clinical efficacy even in the heavily pretreated patients who
progressed on both osimertinib and chemotherapy (ORR 32% in patients with
third- or fourth-line therapy, ORR 13% in patients with fifth-line therapy) [118].
   Antibody drug conjugates (ADCs) are also being employed to overcome
TKI resistance. ADCs are engineered monoclonal antibodies covalently
bound to a cytotoxic drug via a chemical linker to mediate targeted drug

delivery by binding to specific tumor cell surface antigens. After binding, ADCs are internalized via antigen-mediated endocytosis and then undergo lysosomal degradation. The bound cytotoxic drug is released in tumor cells and induces cell apoptosis by exerting cytotoxic effects [119, 120]. For example, MRG003, a novel human IgG_1 anti-EGFR monoclonal antibody conjugated to a monomethyl auristatin E (MMAE), is being evaluated in the phase II study for the efficacy and safety in patients with *EGFR*-positive refractory NSCLC (NCT04838548). Telisotuzumab vedotin (ABBV-399; tel-iso-v), an anti-cMET antibody drug conjugate that has already demonstrated efficacy in advanced NSCLC with cMET overexpression, is being studied in combination with osimertinib in patients with *EGFR* mutations who progressed on osimertinib (NCT02099058) [121]. The novel ERBB3/HER3 antibody–drug conjugate patritumab deruxtecan has shown early limited activity in multiple osimertinib-resistance cases [122] and a large confirmatory phase II trial (HERTHENA-Lung01) [123] has been launched to establish the clinical efficacy and tolerability of this approach. Following favorable early trial results from the phase I dose escalation and expansion study, the FDA approved patritumab deruxtecan as a breakthrough therapy designation for patients with *EGFR*-mutant NSCLC who progressed after third-generation TKI and chemotherapy [122, 124].

In addition to the study of companion agents to overcome TKI resistance, additional TKIs are also being developed. A fourth-generation oral TKI, BLU-945, has demonstrated potent preclinical activity against triple-mutant *EGFR* NSCLC (Exon 19 deletion or L858 R, acquired T790M, and C797S) in xenograft models derived from patients who progressed on multiple lines of treatment [125]. BLU-945 has also demonstrated superior efficacy in tumor regression when combined with gefitinib or osimertinib, and has also been shown to penetrate to the CNS [125]. This triple-mutant EGFR TKI is being studied in a multicenter phase 1/2 study (NCT04862780) in patients with *EGFR*-mutant (T790M, C797S) NSCLC who progressed on prior TKI. It is anticipated that within the next two to five years the aforementioned clinical trial portfolio described in Supplementary Table 1 will result in practice-changing approaches to either delay or manage resistance to the third-generation EGFR TKI osimertinib.

8 Uncommon *EGFR*-Activating Mutations

Other uncommon mutations include point mutations at amino acids in Exon 18 (G719X), 20 (S768I), and 21 (L861Q) [31]. In January, 2018, afatinib was granted expanded access as first-line treatment for the uncommon mutations,

Exon 18 (G719X), 20 (S768I), and 21 (L861Q), after demonstrating efficacy of up to 66% in these less common EGFR subsets [40]. A recent pooled analysis also demonstrated afatinib's efficacy in compound *EGFR* mutations in treatment-naïve and pretreated patients, certain Exon 20 insertions, and uncommon Exon 18 mutations, pointing to afatinib as a potential treatment option for patients with less common mutations [41]. Like afatinib, osimertinib has also been shown to be efficacious for the uncommon mutations, Exon 18 (G719X), Exon 21 (L861Q), and Exon 20 (S768I), as demonstrated in a phase II trial which showed ORR 50% and a median PFS of 8.2 months (95% CI 5.9–10.5 months) [42]. Osimertinib's efficacy in compound mutations has also been reported but has not yet been prospectively studied [126].

9 Immunotherapy in Metastatic *EGFR*-Mutant NSCLC

Checkpoint inhibitors have demonstrated durable and superior OS as monotherapy or as combination chemoimmunotherapy compared to chemotherapy alone in patients with advanced nonsquamous and squamous cell lung cancers [127, 128, 129, 130, 131, 132, 133T, 134]. Patients with *EGFR* mutations, however, were excluded from these studies (KEYNOTE-024, KEYNOTE-189, KEYNOTE-407, KEYNOTE-042) based on inferior outcomes with immunotherapy in *EGFR*-mutant patients in the treatment-naïve or relapsed setting, including with pembro-lizumab (KEYNOTE-001, KEYNOTE-010), nivolumab (CheckMate-057), and atezolizumab (OAK) [135, 136, 137, 138, 139]. A meta-analysis in fact demon-strated a trend toward worse OS (HR 1.11, 95% CI, 0.8–1.53) compared to docetaxel when immunotherapy was used in the relapsed setting in metastatic *EGFR*-mutant NSCLC, and an international retrospective analysis of immune checkpoint inhibitors in advanced NSCLC patients with oncogenic driver muta-tions demonstrated a median PFS of only 2.1 months in the *EGFR*-mutant subgroup [140, 141]. A prospective phase 2 study evaluating pembrolizumab in the first-line setting in *EGFR*-mutant advanced NSCLC with high PD-L1 expression (inclusion criteria PD-L1 ≥ 1%, with 73% of patients with PD-L1 ≥ 50%) demonstrated a lack of efficacy in all enrolled patients, which led to early trial closure [142]. The IMPower150 study was the only large randomized trial that demonstrated some added benefit of immunotherapy (atezolizumab – A) when used in combination with bevacizumab, carboplatin, and paclitaxel (BCP) (median PFS 9.7 months with ABCP vs. 6.1 months with BCP) in patients with *EGFR*-mutant advanced non-squamous lung cancer [110]. Due to the relatively small number of *EGFR*-mutant cases in this trial the data need to be confirmed [110]. More recently, the phase-3 ORIENT-31 trial demonstrated superior PFS with quadruple therapy that included sintilimab, a monoclonal IgG$_4$ antibody against PD-1, a bevacizumab biosimilar

(IBI305), and a platinum doublet compared to chemotherapy alone in a larger set of advanced *EGFR*-mutant nonsquamous NSCLC who had progressed on one or more prior EGFR TKI, suggesting a potential role of immunotherapy in advanced *EGFR*-mutant NSCLC when used in combination with anti-VEGF therapy and doublet chemotherapy [143]. The PACIFIC trial failed to demonstrate a PFS or OS benefit of adjuvant durvalumab after definitive chemoradiation in patients with *EGFR*-mutant stage III NSCLC, although not powered for definitive conclusions for this subset [144]. The generally poor responses of *EGFR*-mutant lung cancers to immune checkpoint inhibitors may be related either to low tumor mutational burden (TMB) or to a "cold" tumor microenvironment in *EGFR*-mutant NSCLC [145, 146, 147, 148, 149, 150, 151].

In addition to lack of immunotherapy response, increased EGFR-related toxicity has been observed if immunotherapy is given within three months prior to EGFR TKI initiation regardless of PD-L1/PD-1 inhibitor duration [152]. In one retrospective study, metastatic *EGFR*-mutant NSCLC patients treated with PD-L1 inhibitor followed by osimertinib demonstrated severe immune-related adverse events in 6 of 41 of patients, including grade 3 pneumonitis, grade 3 colitis, and grade 4 hepatitis [152]. Combination rather than sequential immunotherapy–TKI regimens have also been studied in the phase III CAURAL study, which randomized previously treated T790M-*EGFR*-mutant NSCLC to osimertinib and durvalumab versus osimertinib alone, but the study was terminated early due to increased incidence of interstitial lung disease–like events in the combination durvalumab and osimertinib arm [153]. Single-agent immunotherapy-based regimens have had poor outcomes in advanced *EGFR*-mutant NSCLC. Now additional studies such as KEYNOTE-789 (NCT03515837) are underway to evaluate the efficacy of combined chemoimmunotherapy in advanced *EGFR*-mutant NSCLC after progression from first-line treatment.

10 Management of CNS Disease and Oligometastatic *EGFR*-Mutant NSCLC

About 30–50% of patients with advanced NSCLC have CNS involvement, with higher frequency observed in patients with *EGFR* driver mutations [154, 155]. Up-front stereotactic radiosurgery (SRS) or consolidation radiotherapy to metastatic CNS lesions prior to EGFR TKI have previously demonstrated superior PFS and OS compared to TKI alone with first-generation TKIs [156, 157, 158, 159]. However, with the introduction of osimertinib, with improved blood-brain barrier (BBB) penetration [61, 160, 161, 162, 163, 164, 165, 166, 167], osimertinib has remained the mainstay of treatment in metastatic *EGFR*-mutant

NSCLC with CNS involvement, and the role of up-front SRS remains unclear and remains to be evaluated (NCT03497767) [168]. For patients with residual oligometastatic CNS disease, consolidation radiotherapy may demonstrate improved PFS [169]. For patients who develop CNS progression while on EGFR TKI therapy, SRS, or alternatively, surgical resection followed by SRS, may be appropriate while systemic therapy is continued, as observed with earlier EGFR TKI [23, 170, 171, 172, 173, 174, 175, 176]. For patients who are not candidates for SRS or surgical resection, dexamethasone and supportive care may be appropriate [177]. For those with symptomatic CNS disease, up-front SRS may be appropriate if immediate symptom control is warranted or if there is a delay in access to EGFR TKI therapy [23]. In patients with Exon 20 insertion mutation, mobocertinib, an oral EGFR TKI, has demonstrated CNS activity [178]. Amivantamab-vmjw, also approved in the second-line setting for Exon 20 insertion mutation, however, does not penetrate the BBB, but when used in combination with lazertinib, an oral EGFR TKI targeting Exon 19 deletion, L858 R, and T790M, has been shown to improve ORR and decrease the risk of CNS progression, compared to amivantamab-vmjw monotherapy [37, 118, 179]. For patients with oligometastatic metastases involving non-CNS lesions who do not progress on systemic treatment, definitive local consolidation therapy with stereotactic ablative radiation therapy (SABR) or surgery to the oligometastatic site has been demonstrated to prolong PFS and OS compared to maintenance systemic therapy or observation alone [180] and is the recommended management while continuing systemic treatment. The NORTHSTAR study (NCT03410043) is evaluating the role of the addition of local therapy to osimertinib in advanced *EGFR*-NSCLC.

11 ctDNA in *EGFR*-Mutant NSCLC

Circulating tumor DNA (ctDNA) is widely utilized as a noninvasive diagnostic tool for detecting somatic tumor mutations, especially in the metastatic setting, where there is high tumor burden and increased probability of tumor shedding through tumor necrosis and apoptosis (**Figure 3**). Detection of *EGFR*-mutation through ctDNA and its high concordance with tissue-based assays have been demonstrated in earlier studies, with concordance rates reported to be as high as > 90% and sensitivity and specificity up to 75% and 98%, respectively, with increased sensitivities observed with greater tumor burden [181, 182, 183, 184]. Multiple platforms, including digital (droplet digital polymerase chain reaction (ddPCR), BEAMing PCR) and non-digital assays (cobas® *EGFR* Mutation Test v2, therascreen EGFR amplification refractory mutation system (ARMS) assay), have been developed, with the digital platforms and NGS (next-generation

Applications of ctDNA in *EGFR*-mutant NSCLC

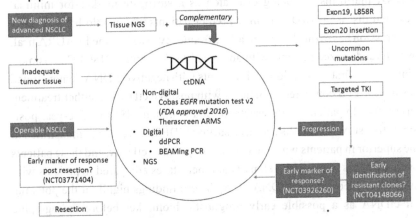

Figure 3 Multiple applications of ctDNA in EGFR-mutant NSCLC in the de novo, metastatic, early stage, and progressive settings.

Notes: NSCLC = non small cell lung cancer.
TKI = tyroskine kinase inhibitor.
ARMS = amplification refractory mutation system.
ddPCR = droplet digital PCR.
BEAMing = beads, emulsions, amplification, and magnetics.
NGS = next-generation sequencing.

sequencing) demonstrating increased sensitivities [184, 185, 186, 187]. The clinical utility of ctDNA as a predictive biomarker to EGFR TKI response was demonstrated in the phase III ENSURE trial, which demonstrated superior PFS with erlotinib compared to chemotherapy in patients who had a positive *EGFR*-mutant ctDNA [188]. This led to the FDA approval of "cobas® EGFR mutation test v2," the first liquid biopsy approved for detection of Exon 19 or L858 R mutations in NSCLC, in June, 2016 [189]. In addition to the easy accessibility of blood-based testing, ctDNA testing allows for a more rapid evaluation of *EGFR* driver mutation, within one week, than tissue-based testing, which may take up to several weeks, and may identify driver mutations that are negative on tissue biopsy due to sampling heterogeneity [190, 191, 192, 193].

ctDNA has also played a clinically significant role in detection of less common mutations. In patients treated with first-generation TKIs who developed acquired T790 M–resistant mutations, plasma and tissue concordance of T790M was reported to be approximately 50% [184, 185, 186]. Higher correlation has been observed with patients with extrathoracic involvement, highlighting again the increased sensitivity of liquid biopsies in settings of increased tumor burden [184, 190, 193]. ctDNA detection of T790M is also a predictive biomarker response to osimertinib [184, 192]. At present, novel ctDNA platforms are being evaluated as a surrogate marker for minimal residual disease (MRD) and may predict patients who would have an early progression based on changes in allele frequency [108]. In the FLAURA trial, which randomized patients with advanced *EGFR*-mutant NSCLC to osimertinib versus first-generation TKI, patients with negative ctDNA demonstrated a superior PFS compared to patients with positive ctDNA in either treatment arm [194]. In patients with resectable *EGFR*-mutant NSCLC, five-year postoperative survival and disease-free survival (DFS) were also demonstrated to be superior in patients with a negative preoperative ctDNA, and these patients were also less likely to develop distant metastases compared to patients with a positive preoperative ctDNA [195]. These findings highlight the potential of ctDNA as a possible early prognostic biomarker before radiographic response.

Current limitations of ctDNA include the existence of multiple platforms, which have variable sensitivities, and suboptimal sensitivity of, at best, 85% in detecting *EGFR*-mutation compared to standard tissue-based assays [187]. Despite these limitations, ctDNA has been widely accepted as a diagnostic tool in identifying *EGFR* driver mutations in the de novo and acquired resistance settings, especially when the risk of biopsy outweighs the benefit or when the initial pathology sample is inadequate [187]. Clinical trials are underway to evaluate whether changes in ctDNA can serve as early predictive markers of response in the metastatic setting (NCT03926260), as markers for early relapse in operable NSCLC (NCT03771404), and as markers to evaluate whether a "track and treat" methodology of temporary treatment of resistant clones detected by continuous monitoring of ctDNA can be utilized in the metastatic setting (NCT04148066).

12 Guidelines and Recommendations for *EGFR*-Mutant NSCLC

Treatment of *EGFR*-mutant NSCLC has made significant progress and represents one of the best examples of the success of precision oncology. Further studies are needed to better understand poor outcomes with immunotherapy in *EGFR*-mutant NSCLC, the role of EGFR TKI in the adjuvant setting following definitive chemoradiation, EGFR TKI in the neoadjuvant setting, combination treatments with anti-VEGF and with chemotherapy, and ctDNA as a prognostic marker for early treatment response in both the adjuvant and metastatic settings. Guidelines recommend tissue-based molecular testing for *EGFR* mutations in stage IB–IIIA surgical biopsies and stage IV patients with adenocarcinoma or squamous cell carcinoma if no or light smoking history, though ctDNA is also widely accepted as an alternative to biomarker testing if tissue biopsy is not feasible or is inadequate in both the de novo and acquired resistance settings [23]. Patients with common *EGFR* mutations (Exon 19 deletion, L858 R) who progress on frontline osimertinib if local and/or asymptomatic may proceed with definitive local treatment with surgery or SRS and can be continued on osimertinib. For patients with Exon 20 insertion mutations, amivantamab-vmjw or mobocertinib, which also have CNS activity, are subsequent treatment options after failure of systemic treatment. In the adjuvant setting, *EGFR*-mutant high-risk stage IB–IIA and stage IIB–IIIA NSCLC should be considered for adjuvant osimertinib, while OS data is eagerly awaited. For metastatic patients who progress on osimertinib, ctDNA or rebiopsy is recommended to evaluate for resistance mechanisms, including off-target bypass mechanisms, on-target acquired mutations, and histologic transformation, with recommendations for clinical trial referral for potential combination-based treatment options with rapidly emerging novel therapeutic options further broadening the horizons and optimizing outcomes in this key disease entity.

References

1. Carpenter, G., L. King, Jr., and S. Cohen, *Epidermal growth factor stimulates phosphorylation in membrane preparations in vitro.* Nature, 1978. **276**(5686): pp. 409–10.

2. Lemmon, M. A. and J. Schlessinger, *Cell signaling by receptor tyrosine kinases.* Cell, 2010. **141**(7): pp. 1117–34.

3. Zhang, X., et al., *An allosteric mechanism for activation of the kinase domain of epidermal growth factor receptor.* Cell, 2006. **125**(6): pp. 1137–49.

4. Li, N., et al., *Guanine-nucleotide-releasing factor hSos1 binds to Grb2 and links receptor tyrosine kinases to Ras signalling.* Nature, 1993. **363**(6424): pp. 85–8.

5. Gale, N. W., et al., *Grb2 mediates the EGF-dependent activation of guanine nucleotide exchange on Ras.* Nature, 1993. **363**(6424): pp. 88–92.

6. Harmer, S. L. and A. L. DeFranco, *Shc contains two Grb2 binding sites needed for efficient formation of complexes with SOS in B lymphocytes.* Mol Cell Biol, 1997. **17**(7): pp. 4087–95.

7. Uribe, M. L., I. Marrocco, and Y. Yarden, *EGFR in cancer: Signaling mechanisms, drugs, and acquired resistance.* Cancers (Basel), 2021. **13**(11): 2748.

8. Wee, P. and Z. Wang, *Epidermal growth factor receptor cell proliferation signaling pathways.* Cancers (Basel), 2017. **9**(5): 52.

9. Mohrherr, J., et al., *STAT3: Versatile functions in non-small cell lung cancer.* Cancers (Basel), 2020. **12**(5): 107.

10. Costa, D. B., et al., *BIM mediates EGFR tyrosine kinase inhibitor-induced apoptosis in lung cancers with oncogenic EGFR mutations.* PLoS Med, 2007. **4**(10): pp. 1669–79; discussion p. 1680.

11. Kobayashi, S., et al., *Transcriptional profiling identifies cyclin D1 as a critical downstream effector of mutant epidermal growth factor receptor signaling.* Cancer Res, 2006. **66**(23): pp. 11389–98.

12. Zhang, Z., et al., *Dual specificity phosphatase 6 (DUSP6) is an ETS-regulated negative feedback mediator of oncogenic ERK signaling in lung cancer cells.* Carcinogenesis, 2010. **31**(4): pp. 577–86.

13. Owens, D. M. and S. M. Keyse, *Differential regulation of MAP kinase signalling by dual-specificity protein phosphatases.* Oncogene, 2007. **26**(22): pp. 3203–13.

14. Chitale, D., et al., *An integrated genomic analysis of lung cancer reveals loss of DUSP4 in EGFR-mutant tumors.* Oncogene, 2009. **28**(31): pp. 2773–83.

15. Shi, Y., et al., *A prospective, molecular epidemiology study of EGFR mutations in Asian patients with advanced non-small-cell lung cancer of adenocarcinoma histology (PIONEER).* J Thorac Oncol, 2014. **9**(2): pp. 154–62.

16. Hirsch, F. R. and P. A. Bunn, Jr., *EGFR testing in lung cancer is ready for prime time.* Lancet Oncol, 2009. **10**(5): pp. 432–3.

17. Zhang, Y. L., et al., *The prevalence of EGFR mutation in patients with non-small cell lung cancer: A systematic review and meta-analysis.* Oncotarget, 2016. **7**(48): pp. 78985–93.

18. Marcoux, N., et al., *EGFR-mutant adenocarcinomas that transform to small-cell lung cancer and other neuroendocrine carcinomas: Clinical outcomes.* J Clin Oncol, 2019. **37**(4): pp. 278–85.

19. Paik, P. K., et al., *Response to erlotinib in patients with EGFR mutant advanced non-small cell lung cancers with a squamous or squamous-like component.* Mol Cancer Ther, 2012. **11**(11): pp. 2535–40.

20. Planchard, D., et al., *Metastatic non-small cell lung cancer: ESMO Clinical Practice Guidelines for diagnosis, treatment and follow-up.* Ann Oncol, 2018. **29**(Suppl. 4): pp. iv192–iv237.

21. Planchard, D., et al., *Clinical Practice Living Guidelines – Metastatic Non-Small-Cell Lung Cancer.* ESMO Guidelines 2020 [cited November 14, 2021]; www.esmo.org/guidelines/lung-and-chest-tumours/clinical-practice-living-guidelines-metastatic-non-small-cell-lung-cancer.

22. D'Angelo, S. P., et al., *Incidence of EGFR exon 19 deletions and L858 R in tumor specimens from men and cigarette smokers with lung adenocarcinomas.* J Clin Oncol, 2011. **29**(15): pp. 2066–70.

23. National Comprehensive Cancer Network (NCCN), *Non-Small Cell Lung Cancer.* October 29, 2021 [cited November 14]; Version 7.2021; www.nccn.org/professionals/physician_gls/pdf/nscl.pdf.

24. Sharma, S. V., et al., *Epidermal growth factor receptor mutations in lung cancer.* Nat Rev Cancer, 2007. **7**(3): pp. 169–81.

25. Hirsch, F. R., et al., *Epidermal growth factor receptor in non-small-cell lung carcinomas: Correlation between gene copy number and protein expression and impact on prognosis.* J Clin Oncol, 2003. **21**(20): pp. 3798–807.

26. Testa, J. R. and J. M. Siegfried, *Chromosome abnormalities in human non-small cell lung cancer.* Cancer Res, 1992. **52**(9 Suppl.): pp. 2702s–2706s.

27. Herbst, R. S., J. V. Heymach, and S. M. Lippman, *Lung cancer.* N Engl J Med, 2008. **359**(13): pp. 1367–80.

28. Yun, C. H., et al., *Structures of lung cancer-derived EGFR mutants and inhibitor complexes: Mechanism of activation and insights into differential inhibitor sensitivity.* Cancer Cell, 2007. **11**(3): pp. 217–27.

29. Maemondo, M., et al., *Gefitinib or chemotherapy for non-small-cell lung cancer with mutated EGFR.* N Engl J Med, 2010. **362**(25): pp. 2380–8.

30. Sequist, L. V., et al., *Phase III study of afatinib or cisplatin plus pemetrexed in patients with metastatic lung adenocarcinoma with EGFR mutations.* J Clin Oncol, 2013. **31**(27): pp. 3327–34.

31. Kobayashi, Y. and T. Mitsudomi, *Not all epidermal growth factor receptor mutations in lung cancer are created equal: Perspectives for individualized treatment strategy.* Cancer Sci, 2016. **107**(9): pp. 1179–86.

32. Riess, J. W., et al., *Diverse EGFR Exon 20 insertions and co-occurring molecular alterations identified by comprehensive genomic profiling of NSCLC.* J Thorac Oncol, 2018. **13**(10): pp. 1560–8.

33. Vasconcelos, P., et al., *EGFR-A763_Y764insFQEA is a unique exon 20 insertion mutation that displays sensitivity to approved and in-development lung cancer EGFR tyrosine kinase inhibitors.* JTO Clin Res Rep, 2020. **1**(3): 100051.

34. Yasuda, H., et al., *Structural, biochemical, and clinical characterization of epidermal growth factor receptor (EGFR) exon 20 insertion mutations in lung cancer.* Sci Transl Med, 2013. **5**(216): 216ra177.

35. Du, Z., et al., *Structure-function analysis of oncogenic EGFR kinase domain duplication reveals insights into activation and a potential approach for therapeutic targeting.* Nat Commun, 2021. **12**(1): 1382.

36. Russo, A., et al., *Heterogeneous responses to epidermal growth factor receptor (EGFR) tyrosine kinase inhibitors (TKIs) in patients with uncommon EGFR mutations: New insights and future perspectives in this complex clinical scenario.* Int J Mol Sci, 2019. **20**(6): 1431.

37. Park, K., et al., *Amivantamab in EGFR exon 20 insertion-mutated non-small-cell lung cancer progressing on platinum chemotherapy: Initial results from the CHRYSALIS phase I study.* J Clin Oncol, 2021. **39**(30): pp. 3391–402.

38. Park, K., et al., *Amivantamab (JNJ-61186372), an anti-EGFR-MET bispecific antibody, in patients with EGFR exon 20 insertion (exon20ins)-mutated non-small cell lung cancer (NSCLC)* [abstract]. J Clin Oncol, 2020. **38**(Suppl.): 9512.

39. Ramalingam, S. S., et al., *Mobocertinib (TAK-788) in EGFR exon 20 insertion (ex20ins)+ metastatic NSCLC (mNSCLC): Additional results from platinum-pretreated patients (pts) and EXCLAIM cohort of phase 1/2 study.* J Clin Oncol, 2021. **39**(15_suppl.): 9014.

40. Yang, J. C., et al., *Clinical activity of afatinib in patients with advanced non-small-cell lung cancer harbouring uncommon EGFR mutations:*

A combined post-hoc analysis of LUX-Lung 2, LUX-Lung 3, and LUX-Lung 6. Lancet Oncol, 2015. **16**(7): pp. 830–8.

41. Yang, J. C., et al., *Afatinib for the treatment of NSCLC harboring uncommon EGFR mutations: A database of 693 cases.* J Thorac Oncol, 2020. **15**(5): pp. 803–15.

42. Cho, J. H., et al., *Osimertinib for patients with non-small-cell lung cancer harboring uncommon EGFR mutations: A multicenter, open-label, phase II trial (KCSG-LU15-09).* J Clin Oncol, 2020. **38**(5): pp. 488–95.

43. Morin, M. J., *From oncogene to drug: Development of small molecule tyrosine kinase inhibitors as anti-tumor and anti-angiogenic agents.* Oncogene, 2000. **19**(56): pp. 6574–83.

44. Mok, T. S., et al., *Gefitinib or carboplatin–paclitaxel in pulmonary adeno-carcinoma.* N Engl J Med, 2009. **361**(10): pp. 947–57.

45. Inoue, A., et al., *Updated overall survival results from a randomized phase III trial comparing gefitinib with carboplatin–paclitaxel for chemo-naïve non-small cell lung cancer with sensitive EGFR gene mutations (NEJ002).* Ann Oncol, 2013. **24**(1): pp. 54–9.

46. Yoshioka, H., et al., *Final overall survival results of WJTOG3405, a randomized phase III trial comparing gefitinib versus cisplatin with docetaxel as the first-line treatment for patients with stage IIIB/IV or postoperative recurrent EGFR mutation-positive non-small-cell lung cancer.* Ann Oncol, 2019. **30**(12): pp. 1978–84.

47. Mitsudomi, T., et al., *Gefitinib versus cisplatin plus docetaxel in patients with non-small-cell lung cancer harbouring mutations of the epidermal growth factor receptor (WJTOG3405): An open label, randomised phase 3 trial.* Lancet Oncol, 2010. **11**(2): pp. 121–8.

48. Fukuoka, M., et al., *Biomarker analyses and final overall survival results from a phase III, randomized, open-label, first-line study of gefitinib versus carboplatin/paclitaxel in clinically selected patients with advanced non-small-cell lung cancer in Asia (IPASS).* J Clin Oncol, 2011. **29**(21): pp. 2866–74.

49. Douillard, J. Y., et al., *First-line gefitinib in Caucasian EGFR mutation-positive NSCLC patients: A phase-IV, open-label, single-arm study.* Br J Cancer, 2014. **110**(1): pp. 55–62.

50. Zhou, C., et al., *Erlotinib versus chemotherapy as first-line treatment for patients with advanced EGFR mutation-positive non-small-cell lung cancer (OPTIMAL, CTONG-0802): A multicentre, open-label, randomised, phase 3 study.* Lancet Oncol, 2011. **12**(8): pp. 735–42.

51. Rosell, R., et al., *Erlotinib versus standard chemotherapy as first-line treatment for European patients with advanced EGFR mutation-positive*

non-small-cell lung cancer (EURTAC): A multicentre, open-label, random-ised phase 3 trial. Lancet Oncol, 2012. **13**(3): pp. 239–46.

52. Patil, V. M., et al., *Phase III study of gefitinib or pemetrexed with carbo-platin in EGFR-mutated advanced lung adenocarcinoma.* ESMO Open, 2017. **2**(1): e000168.

53. Kobayashi, S., et al., *EGFR mutation and resistance of non-small-cell lung cancer to gefitinib.* N Engl J Med, 2005. **352**(8): pp. 786–92.

54. Kosaka, T., et al., *Analysis of epidermal growth factor receptor gene mutation in patients with non-small cell lung cancer and acquired resistance to gefitinib.* Clin Cancer Res, 2006. **12**(19): pp. 5764–9.

55. Solca, F., et al., *Target binding properties and cellular activity of afatinib (BIBW 2992), an irreversible ErbB family blocker.* J Pharmacol Exp Ther, 2012. **343**(2): pp. 342–50.

56. Hsu, W. H., et al., *Overview of current systemic management of EGFR-mutant NSCLC.* Ann Oncol, 2018. **29**(Suppl. 1): pp. i3–i9.

57. Wu, Y. L., et al., *Afatinib versus cisplatin plus gemcitabine for first-line treatment of Asian patients with advanced non-small-cell lung cancer harbouring EGFR mutations (LUX-Lung 6): An open-label, randomised phase 3 trial.* Lancet Oncol, 2014. **15**(2): pp. 213–22.

58. Yang, J. C., et al., *Afatinib versus cisplatin-based chemotherapy for EGFR mutation-positive lung adenocarcinoma (LUX-Lung 3 and LUX-Lung 6): Analysis of overall survival data from two randomised, phase 3 trials.* Lancet Oncol, 2015. **16**(2): pp. 141–51.

59. Mok, T. S., et al., *Improvement in overall survival in a randomized study that compared dacomitinib with gefitinib in patients with advanced non-small-cell lung cancer and EGFR-activating mutations.* J Clin Oncol, 2018. **36**(22): pp. 2244–50.

60. Cross, D. A., et al., *AZD9291, an irreversible EGFR TKI, overcomes T790M-mediated resistance to EGFR inhibitors in lung cancer.* Cancer Discov, 2014. **4**(9): pp. 1046–61.

61. Soria, J. C., et al., *Osimertinib in untreated EGFR-mutated advanced non-small-cell lung cancer.* N Engl J Med, 2018. **378**(2): pp. 113–25.

62. Yang, J. C., et al., *Osimertinib in pretreated T790M-positive advanced non-small-cell lung cancer: AURA Study Phase II Extension Component.* J Clin Oncol, 2017. **35**(12): pp. 1288–96.

63. Goss, G., et al., *Osimertinib for pretreated EGFR Thr790 Met-positive advanced non-small-cell lung cancer (AURA2): A multicentre, open-label, single-arm, phase 2 study.* Lancet Oncol, 2016. **17**(12): pp. 1643–52.

64. Akamatsu, H., et al., *Osimertinib in Japanese patients with EGFR T790M mutation-positive advanced non-small-cell lung cancer: AURA3 trial.* Cancer Sci, 2018. **109**(6): pp. 1930–8.

65. Ramalingam, S. S., et al., *Overall survival with osimertinib in untreated, EGFR-mutated advanced NSCLC.* N Engl J Med, 2020. **382**(1): pp. 41–50.

66. Cho, B., et al., *1258O Amivantamab (JNJ-61186372), an EGFR-MET bispecific antibody, in combination with lazertinib, a 3rd-generation tyrosine kinase inhibitor (TKI), in advanced EGFR NSCLC.* Ann Oncol, 2020. **31**: p. S813.

67. Lu, S., et al., *Randomized phase III trial of aumolertinib (HS-10296, Au) versus gefitinib (G) as first-line treatment of patients with locally advanced or metastatic non-small cell lung cancer (NSCLC) and EGFR exon 19 del or L858 R mutations (EGFRm).* J Clin Oncol, 2021. **39**(15_suppl.): 9013.

68. Nagasaka, M., et al., *Beyond osimertinib: The development of third-generation EGFR tyrosine kinase inhibitors for advanced EGFR+ NSCLC.* J Thorac Oncol, 2021. **16**(5): pp. 740–63.

69. Zhou, Q., et al., *CTONG 1509: Phase III study of bevacizumab with or without erlotinib in untreated Chinese patients with advanced EGFR-mutated NSCLC.* Ann Oncol, 2019. **30**: p. v603.

70. Saito, H., et al., *Erlotinib plus bevacizumab versus erlotinib alone in patients with EGFR-positive advanced non-squamous non-small-cell lung cancer (NEJ026): Interim analysis of an open-label, randomised, multi-centre, phase 3 trial.* Lancet Oncol, 2019. **20**(5): pp. 625–35.

71. Nakagawa, K., et al., *Ramucirumab plus erlotinib in patients with untreated, EGFR-mutated, advanced non-small-cell lung cancer (RELAY): A randomised, double-blind, placebo-controlled, phase 3 trial.* Lancet Oncol, 2019. **20**(12): pp. 1655–69.

72. Le, X., et al., *Dual EGFR-VEGF pathway inhibition: A promising strategy for patients with EGFR-mutant NSCLC.* J Thorac Oncol, 2021. **16**(2): pp. 205–15.

73. Yu, H. A., et al., *Effect of osimertinib and bevacizumab on progression-free survival for patients with metastatic EGFR-mutant lung cancers: A phase 1/2 single-group open-label trial.* JAMA Oncol, 2020. **6**(7): pp. 1048–54.

74. Akamatsu, H., et al., *Efficacy of osimertinib plus bevacizumab vs osimertinib in patients with EGFR T790M-mutated non-small cell lung cancer previously treated with epidermal growth factor receptor-tyrosine kinase inhibitor: West Japan Oncology Group 8715 L Phase 2 randomized clinical trial.* JAMA Oncol, 2021. **7**(3): pp. 386–94.

75. Kenmotsu, H., et al., *Primary results of a randomized phase II study of osimertinib plus bevacizumab versus osimertinib monotherapy for untreated*

patients with non-squamous non-small cell lung cancer harboring EGFR mutations: WJOG9717 L study. Ann Oncol, 2021. **32**: pp. S1283–S1346.

76. Noronha, V., et al., *Gefitinib versus gefitinib plus pemetrexed and carboplatin chemotherapy in EGFR-mutated lung cancer.* J Clin Oncol, 2020. **38**(2): pp. 124–36.

77. Hosomi, Y., et al., *Gefitinib alone versus gefitinib plus chemotherapy for non-small-cell lung cancer with mutated epidermal growth factor receptor: NEJ009 Study.* J Clin Oncol, 2020. **38**(2): pp. 115–23.

78. Wu, Q., et al., *First-generation EGFR-TKI plus chemotherapy versus EGFR-TKI alone as first-line treatment in advanced NSCLC with EGFR activating mutation: A systematic review and meta-analysis of randomized controlled trials.* Front Oncol, 2021. **11**: 598265.

79. Planchard, D., et al., *1401P Osimertinib plus platinum/pemetrexed in newly-diagnosed EGFR mutation (EGFRm)-positive advanced NSCLC: Safety run-in results from the FLAURA2 study.* Ann Oncol, 2020. **31**: p. S888.

80. Kelly, K., et al., *Adjuvant erlotinib versus placebo in patients with stage IB-IIIA non-small-cell lung cancer (RADIANT): A randomized, double-blind, phase III trial.* J Clin Oncol, 2015. **33**(34): pp. 4007–14.

81. Goss, G. D., et al., *Gefitinib versus placebo in completely resected non-small-cell lung cancer: Results of the NCIC CTG BR19 study.* J Clin Oncol, 2013. **31**(27): pp. 3320–6.

82. Wu, Y.-L., et al., *CTONG1104: Adjuvant gefitinib versus chemotherapy for resected N1-N2 NSCLC with EGFR mutation – Final overall survival analysis of the randomized phase III trial 1 analysis of the randomized phase III trial.* American Society of Clinical Oncology, 2020. **38**(15_suppl.): 9005.

83. Wu, Y.-L., et al., *Osimertinib in resected EGFR-mutated non-small-cell lung cancer.* N Engl J Med, 2020. **383**(18): pp. 1711–23.

84. Jorge, S. E., et al., *EGFR exon 20 insertion mutations display sensitivity to Hsp90 inhibition in preclinical models and lung adenocarcinomas.* Clin Cancer Res, 2018. **24**(24): pp. 6548–55.

85. Yasuda, H., S. Kobayashi, and D. B. Costa, *EGFR exon 20 insertion mutations in non-small-cell lung cancer: Preclinical data and clinical implications.* Lancet Oncol, 2012. **13**(1): pp. e23–31.

86. Vasconcelos, P., et al., *Preclinical characterization of mobocertinib highlights the putative therapeutic window of this novel EGFR inhibitor to EGFR exon 20 insertion mutations.* JTO Clin Res Rep, 2021. **2**(3): 100105.

87. Kobayashi, I. S., et al., *EGFR-D770>GY and other rare EGFR exon 20 insertion mutations with a G770 equivalence are sensitive to dacomitinib*

or afatinib and responsive to EGFR exon 20 insertion mutant-active inhibitors in preclinical models and clinical scenarios. Cells, 2021. **10**(12): 3561.

88. Kosaka, T., et al., *Response heterogeneity of EGFR and HER2 exon 20 insertions to covalent EGFR and HER2 inhibitors.* Cancer Res, 2017. **77**(10): pp. 2712–21.

89. Friedlaender, A., et al., *EGFR and HER2 exon 20 insertions in solid tumours: From biology to treatment.* Nat Rev Clin Oncol, 2022. **19**(1): pp. 51–69.

90. Meador, C. B., L. V. Sequist, and Z. Piotrowska, *Targeting EGFR exon 20 insertions in non-small cell lung cancer: Recent advances and clinical updates.* Cancer Discov, 2021. **11**(9): pp. 2145–57.

91. Gonzalvez, F., et al., *Mobocertinib (TAK-788): A targeted inhibitor of egfr exon 20 insertion mutants in non-small cell lung cancer.* Cancer Discov, 2021. **11**(7): pp. 1672–87.

92. Riely, G. J., et al., *Activity and safety of mobocertinib (TAK-788) in previously treated non-small cell lung cancer with EGFR exon 20 insertion mutations from a phase i/ii trial.* Cancer Discov, 2021. **11**(7): pp. 1688–99.

93. Udagawa, H., et al., *TAS6417/CLN-081 is a pan-mutation-selective EGFR tyrosine kinase inhibitor with a broad spectrum of preclinical activity against clinically relevant EGFR mutations.* Mol Cancer Res, 2019. **17**(11): pp. 2233–43.

94. Robichaux, J. P., et al., *Mechanisms and clinical activity of an EGFR and HER2 exon 20-selective kinase inhibitor in non-small cell lung cancer.* Nat Med, 2018. **24**(5): pp. 638–46.

95. Yun, J., et al., *Antitumor activity of amivantamab (JNJ-61186372), an EGFR-MET bispecific antibody, in diverse models of EGFR exon 20 insertion-driven NSCLC.* Cancer Discov, 2020. **10**(8): pp. 1194–209.

96. Vijayaraghavan, S., et al., *Amivantamab (JNJ-61186372), an Fc fnhanced EGFR/cMet bispecific antibody, induces receptor downmodulation and antitumor activity by monocyte/macrophage trogocytosis.* Mol Cancer Ther, 2020. **19**(10): pp. 2044–56.

97. Kobayashi, S., et al., *EGFR mutation and resistance of non–small-cell lung cancer to gefitinib.* N Engl J Med, 2005. **352**(8): pp. 786–92.

98. Nguyen, K.-S. H., S. Kobayashi, and D. B. Costa, *Acquired resistance to epidermal growth factor receptor tyrosine kinase inhibitors in non–small-cell lung cancers dependent on the epidermal growth factor receptor pathway.* Clin Lung Cancer, 2009. **10**(4): pp. 281–9.

99. Niederst, M. J., et al., *RB loss in resistant EGFR mutant lung adenocarcinomas that transform to small-cell lung cancer.* Nature Communications, 2015. **6**(1): 6377.

100. Piper-Vallillo, A. J., L. V. Sequist, and Z. Piotrowska, *Emerging treatment paradigms for EGFR-mutant lung cancers progressing on osimertinib: A review.* J Clin Oncol, 2020: Jco1903123.

101. Pao, W. and J. Chmielecki, *Rational, biologically based treatment of EGFR-mutant non-small-cell lung cancer.* Nat Rev Cancer, 2010. **10**(11): pp. 760–74.

102. Yun, C. H., et al., *The T790M mutation in EGFR kinase causes drug resistance by increasing the affinity for ATP.* Proc Natl Acad Sci USA, 2008. **105**(6): pp. 2070–5.

103. Wu, S.-G. and J.-Y. Shih, *Management of acquired resistance to EGFR TKI–targeted therapy in advanced non-small cell lung cancer.* Mol Cancer, 2018. **17**(1): 38.

104. Ramalingam, S. S., et al., *Overall survival with osimertinib in untreated, EGFR-mutated advanced NSCLC.* N Engl J Med, 2019. **382**(1): pp. 41–50.

105. Passaro, A., et al., *Overcoming therapy resistance in EGFR-mutant lung cancer.* Nat Cancer, 2021. **2**(4): pp. 377–91.

106. Piotrowska, Z. and A. N. Hata, *Resistance to first-line osimertinib in EGFR-mutant NSCLC: Tissue is the issue.* Clin Cancer Res, 2020. **26**(11): pp. 2441–3.

107. Schoenfeld, A. J., et al., *Tumor Analyses Reveal Squamous Transformation and Off-Target Alterations As Early Resistance Mechanisms to First-line Osimertinib in EGFR-Mutant Lung Cancer.* Clin Cancer Res, 2020. **26**(11): pp. 2654–63.

108. Oxnard, G. R., et al., *Assessment of resistance mechanisms and clinical implications in patients with EGFR T790M-positive lung cancer and acquired resistance to osimertinib.* JAMA Oncol, 2018. **4**(11): pp. 1527–34.

109. Socinski, M. A., et al., *Atezolizumab for first-line treatment of metastatic nonsquamous NSCLC.* N Engl J Med, 2018. **378**(24): pp. 2288–301.

110. Reck, M., et al., *1293P IMpower150: Updated efficacy analysis in patients with EGFR mutations.* Ann Oncol, 2020. **31**: pp. S837–S838.

111. Rangachari, D., et al., *EGFR-mutated lung cancers resistant to osimertinib through EGFR C797S respond to first-generation reversible EGFR inhibitors but eventually acquire EGFR T790M/C797S in preclinical models and clinical samples.* J Thorac Oncol, 2019. **14**(11): pp. 1995–2002.

112. Tricker, E. M., et al., *Combined EGFR/MEK inhibition prevents the emergence of resistance in EGFR-mutant lung cancer.* Cancer Discov, 2015. **5**(9): pp. 960–71.

113. Rotow, J. K., et al., *Concurrent osimertinib plus gefitinib for first-line treatment of EGFR-mutated non-small cell lung cancer (NSCLC).* J Clin Oncol, 2020. **38**(15_suppl.): p. 9507.

114. Riely, G., et al., *P1.01-81 phase 3 study of pemetrexed-platinum with or without pembrolizumab for tki-resistant/EGFR-mutated advanced NSCLC: KEYNOTE-789.* J Thorac Oncol, 2018. **13**(10): p. S494.

115. Oxnard, G. R., et al., *TATTON: A multi-arm, phase Ib trial of osimertinib combined with selumetinib, savolitinib, or durvalumab in EGFR-mutant lung cancer.* Ann Oncol, 2020. **31**(4): pp. 507–16.

116. Li, S., et al., *Structural basis for inhibition of the epidermal growth factor receptor by cetuximab.* Cancer Cell, 2005. **7**(4): pp. 301–11.

117. Bauml, J., et al., *Amivantamab in combination with lazertinib for the treatment of osimertinib-relapsed, chemotherapy-naïve EGFR mutant (EGFRm) non-small cell lung cancer (NSCLC) and potential biomarkers for response.* J Clin Oncol, 2021. **39**(15_suppl.): p. 9006.

118. Shu, C. A., et al., *Amivantamab plus lazertinib in post-osimertinib, post-platinum chemotherapy EGFR-mutant non-small cell lung cancer (NSCLC): Preliminary results from CHRYSALIS-2.* Ann Oncol, 2021. **32**: pp. S949–S1039.

119. Chari, R. V., *Targeted cancer therapy: Conferring specificity to cytotoxic drugs.* Acc Chem Res, 2008. **41**(1): pp. 98–107.

120. Beck, A., et al., *Strategies and challenges for the next generation of antibody-drug conjugates.* Nat Rev Drug Discov, 2017. **16**(5): pp. 315–37.

121. Camidge, D. R., et al., *Phase I study of 2- or 3-week dosing of telisotuzumab vedotin, an antibody-drug conjugate targeting c-Met, monotherapy in patients with advanced non-small cell lung carcinoma.* Clin Cancer Res, 2021. **27**(21): pp. 5781–92.

122. Jänne, P. A., et al., *Efficacy and safety of patritumab deruxtecan (HER3-DXd) in EGFR inhibitor-resistant, EGFR-mutated non-small cell lung cancer.* Cancer Discov, 2021. **12**(1): pp. 74–89.

123. Janne, P. A., et al., *HERTHENA-Lung01: A randomized phase 2 study of patritumab deruxtecan (HER3-DXd) in previously treated metastatic EGFR-mutated NSCLC.* J Clin Oncol, 2021. **39**(15_suppl.): TPS9139.

124. Daiichi Sankyo, *Press release: Patritumab Deruxtecan Granted US FDA Breakthrough Therapy Designation in Patients with Metastatic EGFR-Mutated Non-Small Cell Lung Cancer.* 2021; www.daiichisankyo.com/files/news/pressrelease/pdf/202112/20211223_E1.pdf.

125. Schalm, S. S., et al., *1296P BLU-945, a highly potent and selective 4th generation EGFR TKI for the treatment of EGFR T790M/C797S resistant NSCLC.* Ann Oncol, 2020. **31**: p. S839.

126. Rossi, S., et al., *Uncommon single and compound EGFR mutations: Clinical outcomes of a heterogeneous subgroup of NSCLC.* Curr Probl Cancer, 2022. **46**(1): 100787.

127. Reck, M., et al., *Updated analysis of KEYNOTE-024: Pembrolizumab versus platinum-based chemotherapy for advanced non-small-cell lung cancer with PD-L1 tumor proportion score of 50% or greater.* J Clin Oncol, 2019. **37**(7): pp. 537–46.

128. Mok, T. S. K., et al., *Pembrolizumab versus chemotherapy for previously untreated, PD-L1-expressing, locally advanced or metastatic non-small-cell lung cancer (KEYNOTE-042): A randomised, open-label, controlled, phase 3 trial.* Lancet, 2019. **393**(10183): pp. 1819–30.

129. Garassino, M. C., et al., *Patient-reported outcomes following pembrolizumab or placebo plus pemetrexed and platinum in patients with previously untreated, metastatic, non-squamous non-small-cell lung cancer (KEYNOTE-189): A multicentre, double-blind, randomised, placebo-controlled, phase 3 trial.* Lancet Oncol, 2020. **21**(3): pp. 387–97.

130. Gandhi, L., et al., *Pembrolizumab plus chemotherapy in metastatic non-small-cell lung cancer.* N Engl J Med, 2018. **378**(22): pp. 2078–92.

131. Gadgeel, S., et al., *Updated analysis from KEYNOTE-189: Pembrolizumab or placebo plus pemetrexed and platinum for previously untreated metastatic nonsquamous non-small-cell lung cancer.* J Clin Oncol, 2020. **38**(14): pp. 1505–17.

132. Paz-Ares, L., et al., *Pembrolizumab plus chemotherapy for squamous non-small-cell lung cancer.* N Engl J Med, 2018. **379**(21): pp. 2040–51.

133. Paz-Ares, L., et al., *A randomized, placebo-controlled trial of pembrolizumab plus chemotherapy in patients with metastatic squamous NSCLC: Protocol-specified final analysis of KEYNOTE-407.* J Thorac Oncol, 2020. **15**(10): pp. 1657–69.

134. Reck, M., et al., *Pembrolizumab versus chemotherapy for PD-L1-positive non-small-cell lung cancer.* N Engl J Med, 2016. **375**(19): pp. 1823–33.

135. Garon, E. B., et al., *Five-year overall survival for patients with advanced non–small-cell lung cancer treated with pembrolizumab: Results from the phase I KEYNOTE-001 study.* J Clin Oncol, 2019. **37**(28): pp. 2518–27.

136. Herbst, R. S., et al., *Pembrolizumab versus docetaxel for previously treated, PD-L1-positive, advanced non-small-cell lung cancer (KEYNOTE-010): A randomised controlled trial.* Lancet, 2016. **387**(10027): pp. 1540–50.

137. Borghaei, H., et al., *Nivolumab versus docetaxel in advanced nonsquamous non–small-cell lung cancer.* N Engl J Med, 2015. **373**(17): pp. 1627–39.

138. Rittmeyer, A., et al., *Atezolizumab versus docetaxel in patients with previously treated non-small-cell lung cancer (OAK): A phase 3, open-label, multicentre randomised controlled trial.* Lancet, 2017. **389**(10066): pp. 255–65.

139. Rizvi, H., et al., *Molecular determinants of response to anti–programmed cell death (PD)-1 and anti–programmed death-ligand 1 (PD-L1) blockade in patients with non–small-cell lung cancer profiled with targeted next-generation sequencing.* J Clin Oncol, 2018. **36**(7): pp. 633–41.

140. Lee, C. K., et al., *Clinical and molecular characteristics associated with survival among patients treated with checkpoint inhibitors for advanced non–small cell lung carcinoma: A systematic review and meta-analysis.* JAMA Oncol, 2018. **4**(2): pp. 210–16.

141. Mazieres, J., et al., *Immune checkpoint inhibitors for patients with advanced lung cancer and oncogenic driver alterations: Results from the IMMUNOTARGET registry.* Ann Oncol, 2019. **30**(8): pp. 1321–8.

142. Lisberg, A., et al., *A phase ii study of pembrolizumab in EGFR-mutant, PD-L1+, tyrosine kinase inhibitor naive patients with advanced NSCLC.* J Thorac Oncol, 2018. **13**(8): pp. 1138–45.

143. Lu, S., et al., *VP9-2021: ORIENT-31: Phase III study of sintilimab with or without IBI305 plus chemotherapy in patients with EGFR mutated nonsquamous NSCLC who progressed after EGFR-TKI therapy.* Ann Oncol, 2022. **33**(1): pp. 112–3.

144. Antonia, S. J., et al., *Durvalumab after chemoradiotherapy in stage III non–small-cell lung Cancer.* N Engl J Med, 2017. **377**(20): pp. 1919–29.

145. Dong, Z. Y., et al., *EGFR mutation correlates with uninflamed phenotype and weak immunogenicity, causing impaired response to PD-1 blockade in non-small cell lung cancer.* Oncoimmunology, 2017. **6**(11): e1356145.

146. Gainor, J. F., et al., *EGFR mutations and ALK rearrangements are associated with low response rates to PD-1 pathway blockade in non–small cell lung cancer: A retrospective analysis.* Clin Cancer Res, 2016. **22**(18): pp. 4585–93.

147. Budczies, J., et al., *Deciphering the immunosuppressive tumor microenvironment in ALK- and EGFR-positive lung adenocarcinoma.* Cancer Immunol Immunother, 2021. **71**(2): pp. 251–65.

148. Streicher, K., et al., *Increased CD73 and reduced IFNG signature expression in relation to response rates to anti-PD-1(L1) therapies in EGFR-mutant NSCLC.* J Clin Oncol, 2017. **35**(15_suppl.): p. 11505.

149. Park, L. C., et al., *Immunologic and clinical implications of CD73 expression in non-small cell lung cancer (NSCLC).* J Clin Oncol, 2018. **36**(15_suppl.): p. 12050.

150. Passarelli, A., et al., *Targeting immunometabolism mediated by CD73 pathway in EGFR-mutated non-small cell lung cancer: A new hope for overcoming immune resistance.* Front Immunol, 2020. **11**: 1479.

151. Yu, S., et al., *Immunotherapy strategy of EGFR mutant lung cancer.* Am J Cancer Res, 2018. **8**(10): pp. 2106–15.

152. Schoenfeld, A. J., et al., *Severe immune-related adverse events are common with sequential PD-(L)1 blockade and osimertinib.* Ann Oncol, 2019. **30**(5): pp. 839–44.

153. Yang, J. C., et al., *Osimertinib plus durvalumab versus osimertinib monotherapy in EGFR T790M-positive NSCLC following previous EGFR TKI therapy: CAURAL Brief Report.* J Thorac Oncol, 2019. **14**(5): pp. 933–9.

154. Hu, C., et al., *Nonsmall cell lung cancer presenting with synchronous solitary brain metastasis.* Cancer, 2006. **106**(9): pp. 1998–2004.

155. Ge, M., et al., *High probability and frequency of EGFR mutations in non-small cell lung cancer with brain metastases.* J Neurooncol, 2017. **135**(2): pp. 413–18.

156. Soon, Y. Y., et al., *EGFR tyrosine kinase inhibitors versus cranial radiation therapy for EGFR mutant non-small cell lung cancer with brain metastases: A systematic review and meta-analysis.* Radiother Oncol, 2015. **114**(2): pp. 167–72.

157. Magnuson, W. J., et al., *Management of brain metastases in tyrosine kinase inhibitor–naïve epidermal growth factor receptor–mutant non-small-cell lung cancer: A retrospective multi-institutional analysis.* J Clin Oncol, 2017. **35**(10): pp. 1070–7.

158. Xu, Q., et al., *Consolidative local ablative therapy improves the survival of patients with synchronous oligometastatic NSCLC harboring EGFR activating mutation treated with first-line EGFR-TKIs.* J Thorac Oncol, 2018. **13**(9): pp. 1383–92.

159. Wang, X. and M. Zeng, *First-line tyrosine kinase inhibitor with or without aggressive upfront local radiation therapy in patients with EGFRm oligometastatic non-small cell lung cancer: Interim results of a randomized phase III, open-label clinical trial (SINDAS) (NCT02893332).* J Clin Oncol, 2020. **38**(15_suppl.): p. 9508.

160. Ballard, P., et al., *Preclinical comparison of osimertinib with other EGFR-TKIs in EGFR-mutant NSCLC brain metastases models, and early evidence of clinical brain metastases activity.* Clin Cancer Res, 2016. **22**(20): pp. 5130–40.

161. Mok, T. S., et al., *Osimertinib or platinum–pemetrexed in EGFR T790M-positive lung cancer.* N Engl J Med, 2016. **376**(7): pp. 629–40.

162. Goss, G., et al., *CNS response to osimertinib in patients with T790M-positive advanced NSCLC: Pooled data from two phase II trials.* Ann Oncol, 2018. **29**(3): pp. 687–93.

163. Yamaguchi, H., et al., *A phase II study of osimertinib for radiotherapy-naive central nervous system metastasis from NSCLC: Results for the T790M cohort of the OCEAN study (LOGIK1603/WJOG9116 L).* J Thorac Oncol, 2021. **16**(12): pp. 2121–32.

164. Wu, Y.-L., et al., *CNS efficacy of osimertinib in patients with T790M-positive advanced non–small-cell lung cancer: Data from a randomized phase III trial (AURA3).* J Clin Oncol, 2018. **36**(26): pp. 2702–9.

165. Yang, J. C. H., et al., *Osimertinib in patients with epidermal growth factor receptor mutation-positive non-small-cell lung cancer and leptomeningeal metastases: The BLOOM study.* J Clin Oncol, 2020. **38**(6): pp. 538–47.

166. Lee, J., et al., *Osimertinib improves overall survival in patients with EGFR-mutated NSCLC with leptomeningeal metastases regardless of T790M mutational status.* J Thorac Oncol, 2020. **15**(11): pp. 1758–66.

167. Ahn, M.-J., et al., *Osimertinib for patients with leptomeningeal metastases associated with EGFR T790M-positive advanced NSCLC: The AURA leptomeningeal metastases analysis.* J Thorac Oncol, 2020. **15**(4): pp. 637–48.

168. Zhai, X., et al., *Therapeutic effect of osimertinib plus cranial radiotherapy compared to osimertinib alone in NSCLC patients with EGFR-activating mutations and brain metastases: A retrospective study.* Radiat Oncol, 2021. **16**(1): 233.

169. Zeng, Y., et al., *The value of local consolidative therapy in osimertinib-treated non-small cell lung cancer with oligo-residual disease.* Radiat Oncol, 2020. **15**(1): 207.

170. Laurie, S. A., et al., *Canadian consensus: Oligoprogressive, pseudoprogressive, and oligometastatic non-small-cell lung cancer.* Curr Oncol, 2019. **26**(1): pp. e81–e93.

171. Shukuya, T., et al., *Continuous EGFR-TKI administration following radiotherapy for non-small cell lung cancer patients with isolated CNS failure.* Lung Cancer, 2011. **74**(3): pp. 457–61.

172. Weickhardt, A. J., et al., *Local ablative therapy of oligoprogressive disease prolongs disease control by tyrosine kinase inhibitors in oncogene-addicted non-small-cell lung cancer.* J Thorac Oncol, 2012. **7**(12): pp. 1807–14.

173. Di Noia, V., et al., *Treating disease progression with osimertinib in EGFR-mutated non-small-cell lung cancer: Novel targeted agents and combination strategies.* ESMO Open, 2021. **6**(6): 100280.

174. Le, X., et al., *Landscape of EGFR-dependent and -independent resistance mechanisms to osimertinib and continuation therapy beyond progression in EGFR-mutant NSCLC.* Clin Cancer Res, 2018. **24**(24): pp. 6195–203.

175. Mu, Y., et al., *Clinical modality of resistance and subsequent management of patients with advanced non-small cell lung cancer failing treatment with osimertinib.* Target Oncol, 2019. **14**(3): pp. 335–42.

176. Cortellini, A., et al., *Osimertinib beyond disease progression in T790M EGFR-positive NSCLC patients: A multicenter study of clinicians' attitudes.* Clin Transl Oncol, 2020. **22**(6): pp. 844–51.

177. Mulvenna, P., et al., *Dexamethasone and supportive care with or without whole brain radiotherapy in treating patients with non-small cell lung cancer with brain metastases unsuitable for resection or stereotactic radiotherapy (QUARTZ): Results from a phase 3, non-inferiority, randomised trial.* Lancet, 2016. **388**(10055): pp. 2004–14.

178. Zhou, C., et al., *Treatment outcomes and safety of mobocertinib in platinum-pretreated patients with EGFR exon 20 insertion–positive metastatic non–small cell lung cancer: A phase 1/2 open-label nonrandomized clinical trial.* JAMA Oncol, 2021: e214761.

179. Dhillon, S., *Lazertinib: First Approval.* Drugs, 2021. **81**(9): pp. 1107–13.

180. Gomez, D. R., et al., *Local consolidative therapy vs. maintenance therapy or observation for patients with oligometastatic non–small-cell lung cancer: Long-term results of a multi-institutional, phase II, randomized study.* J Clin Oncol, 2019. **37**(18): pp. 1558–65.

181. Douillard, J. Y., et al., *Gefitinib treatment in EGFR mutated caucasian NSCLC: Circulating-free tumor DNA as a surrogate for determination of EGFR status.* J Thorac Oncol, 2014. **9**(9): pp. 1345–53.

182. Wu, Y. L., et al., *Clinical utility of a blood-based EGFR mutation test in patients receiving first-line erlotinib therapy in the ENSURE, FASTACT-2, and ASPIRATION studies.* Lung Cancer, 2018. **126**: pp. 1–8.

183. Qiu, M., et al., *Circulating tumor DNA is effective for the detection of EGFR mutation in non-small cell lung cancer: A meta-analysis.* Cancer Epidemiol Biomarkers Prev, 2015. **24**(1): pp. 206–12.

184. Jenkins, S., et al., *Plasma ctDNA analysis for detection of the EGFR T790M mutation in patients with advanced non-small cell lung cancer.* J Thorac Oncol, 2017. **12**(7): pp. 1061–70.

185. Thress, K. S., et al., *EGFR mutation detection in ctDNA from NSCLC patient plasma: A cross-platform comparison of leading technologies to support the clinical development of AZD9291.* Lung Cancer, 2015. **90**(3): pp. 509–15.

186. Papadimitrakopoulou, V. A., et al., *Epidermal growth factor receptor mutation analysis in tissue and plasma from the AURA3 trial: Osimertinib versus platinum-pemetrexed for T790M mutation-positive advanced non-small cell lung cancer.* Cancer, 2020. **126**(2): pp. 373–80.

187. Rolfo, C., et al., *Liquid biopsy for advanced non-small cell lung cancer (NSCLC): A statement paper from the IASLC.* J Thorac Oncol, 2018. **13**(9): pp. 1248–68.

188. Wu, Y. L., et al., *First-line erlotinib versus gemcitabine/cisplatin in patients with advanced EGFR mutation-positive non-small-cell lung cancer: Analyses from the phase III, randomized, open-label, ENSURE study.* Ann Oncol, 2015. **26**(9): pp. 1883–9.

189. US Food and Drug Administration. *cobas EGFR Mutation Test v2.* June 2, 2016 [cited November 1, 2021]; www.fda.gov/drugs/resources-information-approved-drugs/cobas-egfr-mutation-test-v2.

190. Sacher, A. G., et al., *Prospective validation of rapid plasma genotyping for the detection of EGFR and KRAS mutations in advanced lung cancer.* JAMA Oncol, 2016. **2**(8): pp. 1014–22.

191. Oxnard, G. R., et al., *Association between plasma genotyping and outcomes of treatment with osimertinib (AZD9291) in advanced non-small-cell lung cancer.* J Clin Oncol, 2016. **34**(28): pp. 3375–82.

192. Remon, J., et al., *Osimertinib benefit inEGFR-mutant NSCLC patients withT790M-mutation detected by circulating tumour DNA.* Ann Oncol, 2017. **28**(4): pp. 784–90.

193. Sundaresan, T. K., et al., *Detection of T790M, the acquired resistance EGFR mutation, by tumor biopsy versus noninvasive blood-based analyses.* Clin Cancer Res, 2016. **22**(5): pp. 1103–10.

194. Gray, J. E., et al., *Tissue and plasma EGFR mutation analysis in the FLAURA trial: Osimertinib versus comparator EGFR tyrosine kinase inhibitor as first-line treatment in patients with EGFR-mutated advanced non-small cell lung cancer.* Clin Cancer Res, 2019. **25**(22): pp. 6644–52.

195. Guo, K., et al., *Detection of epidermal growth factor receptor (EGFR) mutations from preoperative circulating tumor DNA (ctDNA) as a prognostic predictor for stage I-III non-small cell lung cancer (NSCLC) patients with baseline tissue EGFR mutations.* Transl Lung Cancer Res, 2021. **10**(7): pp. 3213–25.

Cambridge Elements ☰

Molecular Oncology

Edward P. Gelmann

University of Arizona

Dr. Edward P. Gelmann is John Norton Professor of Prostate Cancer Research at the University of Arizona and the University of Arizona Cancer Center. Dr. Gelmann previously headed Divisions of Hematology/Oncology at both Georgetown University and Columbia University. He has been the recipient of NIH, DOD, and NIEHS grants for his research, which has spanned cancer basic, clinical, and population sciences. Dr. Gelmann's research currently focuses on the early stages of prostate carcinogenesis and the development of novel therapeutics for prostate cancer. He continues to be involved in clinical care and clinical research of genitourinary malignancies. He has an active clinical practice and directs GU clinical research at the Cancer Center. Dr. Gelmann has published extensively and is senior editor of the book *Molecular Oncology: Causes of Cancer and Targets for Treatment* (Cambridge University Press, 2013).

About the Series

Therapeutics in clinical oncology are based increasingly on molecular drivers and hallmarks of cancers. *Elements in Molecular Oncology* provides a timely overview of topics in oncology for researchers and clinicians. By focusing on cancer sites or pathways, this series presents information on the latest findings on cancer causation and treatment.

Cambridge Elements ≡

Molecular Oncology

Elements in the Series

Personalized Drug Screening for Functional Tumor Profiling
Victoria El-Khoury, Tatiana Michel, Hichul Kim, and Yong-Jun Kwon

Therapeutic Targeting of RAS Mutant Cancers
Edward C. Stites, Kendra Paskvan, and Shumei Kato

Targeting Oncogenic Driver Mutations in Lung Cancer
Matthew Lee, Fawzi Abu Rous, Alain Borczuk, Stephen Liu, Shirish Gadgeel, and Balazs Halmos

EGFR-Directed Therapy in Lung Cancer
So Yeon Kim, Daniel B. Costa, Daisuke Shibahara, Susumu Kobayashi, and Balazs Halmos

A full series listing is available at: www.cambridge.org/EMO

Printed in the United States
by Baker & Taylor Publisher Services

Printed in the United States
by Baker & Taylor Publisher Services